THIS BOOK BELONGS TO

. . . .

OBSERVATIONS

MILK

yummy!

1ST MEAL

2ND MEAL

3RD MEAL

SNACKS

OBSERVATIONS

MILK

TIME	AMOUNT

OBSERVATIONS

MILK

yummy!

1ST MEAL

2ND MEAL

3RD MEAL

SNACKS

OBSERVATIONS

MILK

TIME	AMOUNT

MILK

. . . . / . . . . / . . .

yummy!

1ST MEAL

2ND MEAL

3RD MEAL

SNACKS

OBSERVATIONS

MILK

TIME	AMOUNT

OBSERVATIONS

MILK

yummy!

1ST MEAL

OBSERVATIONS

2ND MEAL

3RD MEAL

MILK

TIME	AMOUNT

SNACKS

MILK

.... / .... / ...

yummy!

1ST MEAL

2ND MEAL

3RD MEAL

SNACKS

OBSERVATIONS

MILK

TIME	AMOUNT

MILK

. . . / . . . / . . .

yummy!

1ST MEAL

2ND MEAL

3RD MEAL

SNACKS

OBSERVATIONS

MILK

TIME	AMOUNT

. . . . / . . . . / . . .

yummy!

1ST MEAL

2ND MEAL

3RD MEAL

SNACKS

OBSERVATIONS

MILK

TIME	AMOUNT

OBSERVATIONS

MILK

····/····/···

yummy!

1ST MEAL		OBSERVATIONS

1ST MEAL

2ND MEAL

3RD MEAL

SNACKS

OBSERVATIONS

MILK

TIME	AMOUNT

OBSERVATIONS

MILK

. . . / . . . / . . .

yummy!

1ST MEAL	OBSERVATIONS

2ND MEAL

3RD MEAL

MILK

TIME	AMOUNT

SNACKS

MILK

yummy!

. . . / . . . / . . .

1ST MEAL

2ND MEAL

3RD MEAL

SNACKS

OBSERVATIONS

MILK

TIME	AMOUNT

OBSERVATIONS

MILK

yummy!

. . . . / . . . . / . . .

1ST MEAL

2ND MEAL

3RD MEAL

SNACKS

OBSERVATIONS

MILK

TIME	AMOUNT

OBSERVATIONS

MILK

yummy!

1ST MEAL

2ND MEAL

3RD MEAL

SNACKS

OBSERVATIONS

MILK

TIME	AMOUNT

yummy!

1ST MEAL

2ND MEAL

3RD MEAL

SNACKS

OBSERVATIONS

MILK

TIME	AMOUNT

MILK

... / ... / ...

yummy!

1ST MEAL	**OBSERVATIONS**
2ND MEAL	
3RD MEAL	**MILK**
	TIME AMOUNT
SNACKS	

MILK

yummy!

1ST MEAL

2ND MEAL

3RD MEAL

SNACKS

OBSERVATIONS

MILK

TIME	AMOUNT

OBSERVATIONS

MILK

. . . / . . . . / . . .

yummy!

1ST MEAL	OBSERVATIONS

2ND MEAL

3RD MEAL

MILK

TIME	AMOUNT

SNACKS

MILK

... / ... / ...

yummy!

| 1ST MEAL | OBSERVATIONS |

2ND MEAL

3RD MEAL

MILK

TIME   AMOUNT

SNACKS

OBSERVATIONS

OBSERVATIONS

MILK

... / ... / ...

yummy!

1ST MEAL

2ND MEAL

3RD MEAL

SNACKS

OBSERVATIONS

MILK

TIME	AMOUNT

OBSERVATIONS

MILK

. . . . / . . . . / . . .

yummy!

1ST MEAL

2ND MEAL

3RD MEAL

SNACKS

OBSERVATIONS

MILK

TIME	AMOUNT

OBSERVATIONS

MILK

yummy!

... / ... / ...

1ST MEAL

| 2ND MEAL |

| 3RD MEAL |

| SNACKS |

OBSERVATIONS

MILK

TIME	AMOUNT

MILK

... / ... / ...

yummy!

1ST MEAL

2ND MEAL

3RD MEAL

SNACKS

OBSERVATIONS

MILK

TIME	AMOUNT

OBSERVATIONS

MILK

yummy!

1ST MEAL

2ND MEAL

3RD MEAL

SNACKS

OBSERVATIONS

MILK

TIME	AMOUNT

OBSERVATIONS

MILK

· · · / · · · / · · ·

yummy!

1ST MEAL	OBSERVATIONS

| 2ND MEAL | |

| 3RD MEAL | MILK |

	TIME	AMOUNT

| SNACKS | |

MILK

. . . / . . . / . . .

yummy!

| 1ST MEAL | OBSERVATIONS |

2ND MEAL

3RD MEAL

MILK

TIME   AMOUNT

SNACKS

OBSERVATIONS

MILK

··· / ··· / ···

yummy!

1ST MEAL	**OBSERVATIONS**
2ND MEAL	
3RD MEAL	**MILK**
	TIME AMOUNT
SNACKS	

MILK

yummy!

..... / ..... / .....

1ST MEAL

2ND MEAL

3RD MEAL

SNACKS

OBSERVATIONS

MILK

TIME	AMOUNT

OBSERVATIONS

OBSERVATIONS

MILK

... / ... / ...

yummy!

1ST MEAL

2ND MEAL

3RD MEAL

SNACKS

OBSERVATIONS

MILK

TIME	AMOUNT

OBSERVATIONS

MILK

yummy!

... / ... / ...

1ST MEAL

2ND MEAL

3RD MEAL

SNACKS

OBSERVATIONS

MILK

TIME	AMOUNT

yummy!

1ST MEAL

2ND MEAL

3RD MEAL

SNACKS

OBSERVATIONS

MILK

TIME	AMOUNT

OBSERVATIONS

MILK

yummy!

. . . / . . . / . . .

1ST MEAL

2ND MEAL

3RD MEAL

SNACKS

OBSERVATIONS

MILK

TIME	AMOUNT

OBSERVATIONS

MILK

. . . . / . . . . / . . . .

yummy!

1ST MEAL

2ND MEAL

3RD MEAL

SNACKS

OBSERVATIONS

MILK

TIME	AMOUNT

OBSERVATIONS

MILK

yummy!

1ST MEAL	OBSERVATIONS

2ND MEAL

3RD MEAL

MILK

TIME   AMOUNT

SNACKS

MILK

... / ... / ...

yummy!

1ST MEAL

2ND MEAL

3RD MEAL

SNACKS

OBSERVATIONS

MILK

TIME	AMOUNT

MILK

yummy!

1ST MEAL

2ND MEAL

3RD MEAL

SNACKS

OBSERVATIONS

MILK

TIME	AMOUNT

OBSERVATIONS

MILK

yummy!

1ST MEAL

2ND MEAL

3RD MEAL

SNACKS

OBSERVATIONS

MILK

TIME	AMOUNT

. . . . / . . . . / . . .

yummy!

1ST MEAL	**OBSERVATIONS**
2ND MEAL	
3RD MEAL	**MILK**
	TIME AMOUNT
SNACKS	

OBSERVATIONS

MILK

yummy!

· · · · / · · · · / · · ·

1ST MEAL	OBSERVATIONS
2ND MEAL	
3RD MEAL	**MILK**
	TIME	AMOUNT
SNACKS	

OBSERVATIONS

MILK

....../....../......

yummy!

1ST MEAL	OBSERVATIONS
2ND MEAL	
3RD MEAL	**MILK**
	TIME AMOUNT
SNACKS	

... / ... / ...

yummy!

1ST MEAL

2ND MEAL

3RD MEAL

SNACKS

OBSERVATIONS

MILK

TIME	AMOUNT

MILK

... / ... / ...

yummy!

| 1ST MEAL | OBSERVATIONS |

2ND MEAL

3RD MEAL

MILK

| TIME | AMOUNT |

SNACKS

MILK

yummy!

......./......./......

1ST MEAL

2ND MEAL

3RD MEAL

SNACKS

OBSERVATIONS

MILK

TIME	AMOUNT

yummy!

. . . / . . . / . . .

1ST MEAL

2ND MEAL

3RD MEAL

SNACKS

OBSERVATIONS

MILK

TIME	AMOUNT

OBSERVATIONS

MILK

yummy!

... / .... / ...

1ST MEAL	OBSERVATIONS
2ND MEAL	
3RD MEAL	**MILK**
	TIME AMOUNT
SNACKS	

OBSERVATIONS

MILK

yummy!

1ST MEAL

2ND MEAL

3RD MEAL

SNACKS

OBSERVATIONS

MILK

TIME	AMOUNT

yummy!

. . . . / . . . . / . . .

1ST MEAL

2ND MEAL

3RD MEAL

SNACKS

OBSERVATIONS

MILK

TIME	AMOUNT

OBSERVATIONS

MILK

yummy!

1ST MEAL

2ND MEAL

3RD MEAL

SNACKS

OBSERVATIONS

MILK

TIME	AMOUNT

MILK

yummy!

... / ... / ...

1ST MEAL

2ND MEAL

3RD MEAL

SNACKS

OBSERVATIONS

MILK

TIME	AMOUNT

OBSERVATIONS

MILK

····· / ····· / ···

yummy!

1ST MEAL	**OBSERVATIONS**
2ND MEAL	
3RD MEAL	**MILK**
	TIME — AMOUNT
SNACKS	

..... / ..... / .....

yummy!

| 1ST MEAL | OBSERVATIONS |

2ND MEAL

3RD MEAL

MILK

TIME	AMOUNT

SNACKS

MILK

yummy!

1ST MEAL

2ND MEAL

3RD MEAL

SNACKS

OBSERVATIONS

MILK

TIME	AMOUNT

Printed in Great Britain
by Amazon